Herbs That Cure

Children's Health Problems

Time-Tested Herbal Remedies

No Side-effects

by

Prayank

Contents

Introduction

Children's health problems need special care due to their weak constitution. Also the prescriptions and dosage has to be suitably modified for them. In the book, you will find brief details of herbs that can be used to cure some heath problems specific to children - colic, cough, flatulence, mumps etc.

It also gives you an option to choose the herb that is easily available in your locality. Herb names may be different in different places, hence you should rely on botanical names to find how it is known in a particular place/location.

Though there are people who treat ailments inexpensively with herbal remedies, most consider it as the last minute miracle worker once all other avenues of treatments have been exhausted.

Such an approach discounts the sophisticated and elaborately documented information dealing with specific medicinal applications of herbs for specific complaints. The methods of herbal remedies are designed for optimum beneficial use and tested innumerable times in actual practice.

While every effort has been made to verify the authenticity of information contained in this book, it is not intended as a substitute for medicinal consultation with a physician. The publisher and the author are in no way liable for the use of information contained in the book.

1. Ajwain

(Trachyspermum ammi)

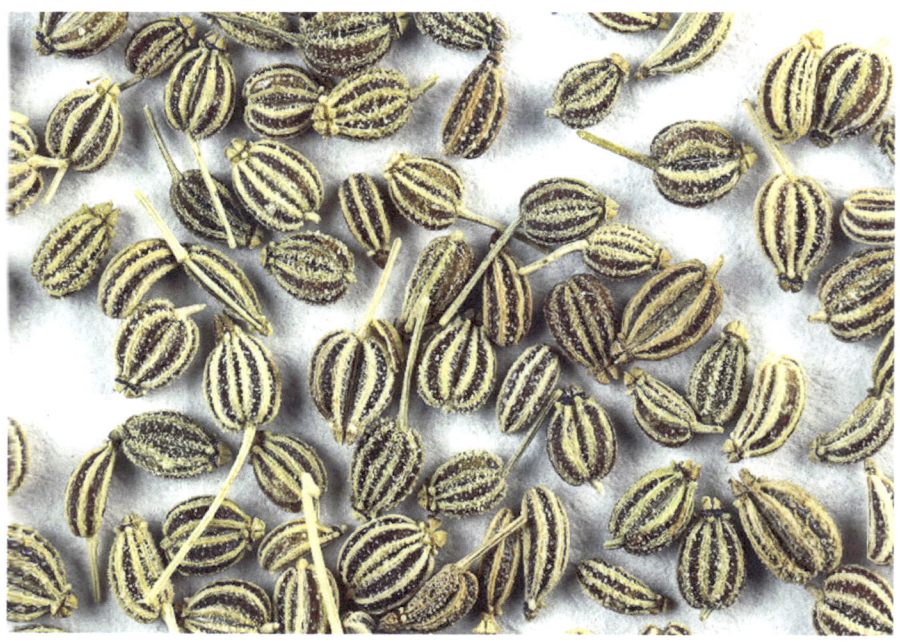

General

Ajwain or ajowan, (also known as bishop's weed, ajowan, caraway, carom seeds, or thymol seeds) is used for the treatment of a number of ailments: dyspepsia, diarrhoea, flatulence, indigestion, spasmodic disorders, microbial infections, etc. It has well-known anti-bacterial properties.

There are two varieties of the plant, ajwain : one with long seeds and the other with short ones. It is the short-seeded variety which is preferred for medicinal use.

Profile

Botanical Name : Trachyspermum ammi

Other Species : Sisan ammi, Carum copticum

Family : Umbelliferae

Appearance : Small, erect, annual herbs with soft fine hairs. Leaves- feather like. Fruits – strong smelling, small, egg-shaped, gray in color.

Medicinal Parts : Fruits (seeds)

Distribution : A plant originated in the Middle East, possibly in Egypt, and the Indian subcontinent, but also in Iran and Afghanistan.

Ailments and Cure

Nasal congestion in children – Crush a fistful of ajwain seeds and tie up in a cotton napkin. Place it near the pillow of the child.

Chest congestion – Add 1 tsp each ajwain seeds and turmeric powder to ½ liter of boiling water. Cool and administer 1 tbsp of this mixture along with 1 tsp honey to the child.

Colic pains, gas problems, gastralgia, indigestion, repeated belching, pain in the abdomen around navel – Grind 2 tsp each ajwain and dried ginger into a fine powder. Add a little black salt. Take 1 tsp of this mixture with 1 teacup warm water frequently. (Note: Avoid solid food intake for better results.)

2. <u>Arkh</u>

(Calotrpis gigantea)

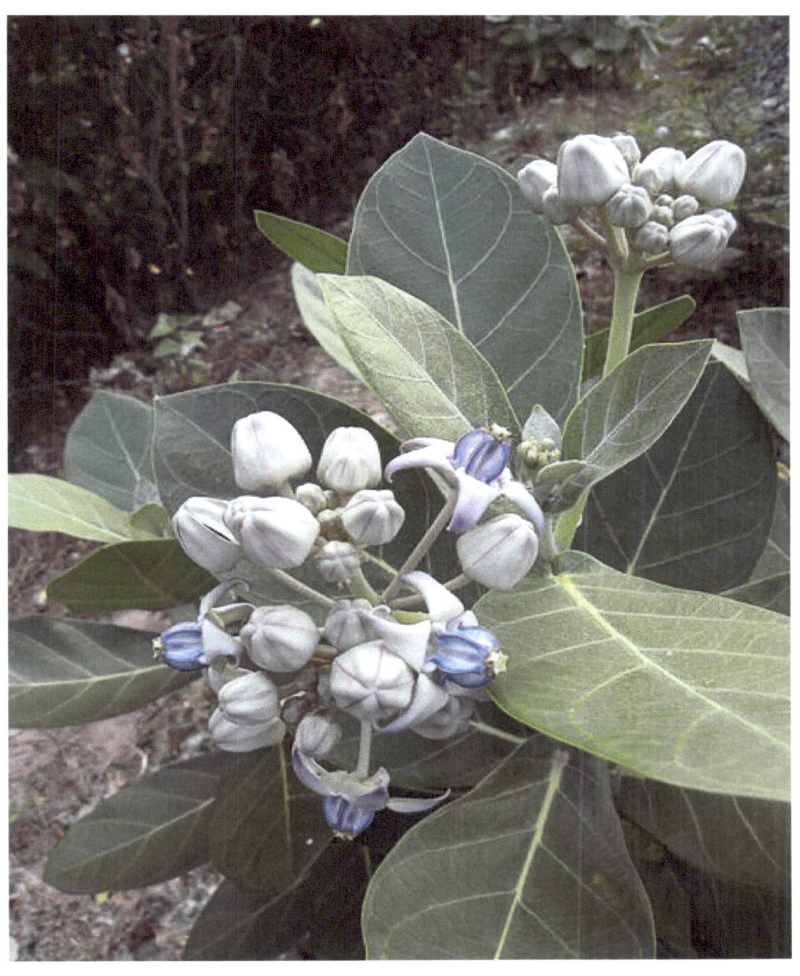

General

Although the plant is attractive to look at and medicinally useful, it gives off a foul smell. The plant blooms round the year. The plant's Sanskrit name refer to its strong, caustic action.

It is a large shrub growing to 4 m tall. It has clusters of waxy flowers that are either white or lavender in colour. Each flower consists of five pointed petals and a small, elegant "crown" rising from the center, which holds the stamens. The plant has oval, light green leaves and milky stem.

Profile

Botanical Name : Calotropis gigantea

Other Species : Calotropis procera

Family : Asclepiadoideae

Appearance : Erect pale greyish shrub covered with white cottony coat. Leaves - simple, ear shaped at base. Flowers - lilac or dull white. Fruits - in pairs, resemble mangoes, containing loose, silky and fibrous growth.

Medicinal Parts : Flowers, latex, leaves, root

Distribution : Native to Cambodia, Indonesia, Malaysia, Philippines, Thailand, Sri Lanka, India and China.

Ailments and Cure

Colic, Gastralsia - Grind 1 tbsp flowers along with 1 tbsp ajwain, 2 tsp dried ginger and 1 tsp black salt. Add a little lime juice and roll into pea - sized pills. Dose : 1 pill with 1 cup hot water.

Enlargement of the abdomen - Lightly roasted leaves are applied locally.

Mumps - Tie the leaves over affected areas.

3. <u>Brahmi</u>

(Bacopa monnieri)

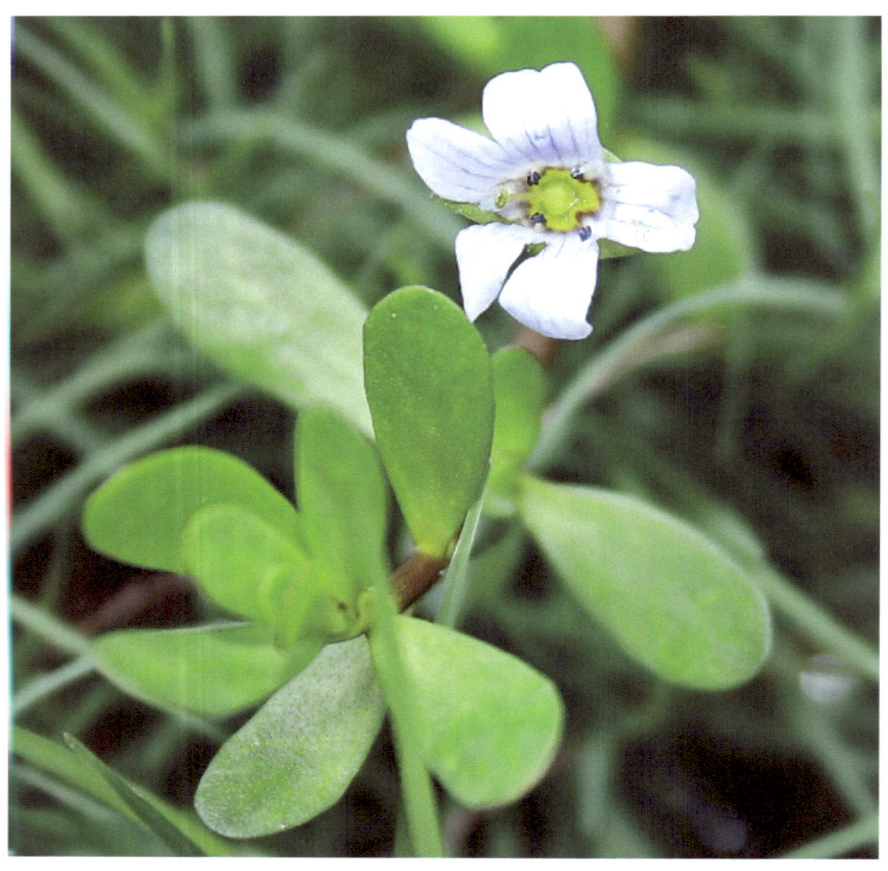

General

A perennial, creeping herb whose habitat includes wetlands and muddy shores. Brahmi is also the name given to mandukparni (Centella asiatica), particularly in north India but they are different herbs.

This herb is usually used for nervous disorders such as insanity, epilepsy, neurasthenia, nervous breakdown etc. The plant contains an alkaloid, related to strychnine, but less toxic and hence capable of safe use by those who want to stimulate the intellect and the faculty of speech. It is also used to strengthen and tone the heart muscles.

Profile

Botanical Name : Bacopa monnieri

Other Species : Herpestis monnieria, Monnieri cuneifolia, Lysimachia monnieri

Family : Fabaceae

Sub-family : Scrophlariaceae

Appearance : A small, prostrate herb with ascending branches. Roots arise on the nodes of stem. Leaves - fleshy, oblong with obscure veins. Flowers - bluish white or lilac. Fruit - egg like with persistent style.

Medicinal Parts : Leaves, fruits, the whole plant

Distribution: It commonly grows in marshy areas throughout India, Nepal, Sri Lanka, China, Taiwan, and Vietnam, and is also found in Florida, Hawaii and other southern states of the USA where it can be grown in damp conditions by the pond or bog garden.

Ailments and Cure

Cough in children - Boil the crushed plant (about 2 cups), make a poultice and place on the chest for half an hour. Repeat till cured.

4. <u>Calamus</u>

(Acorus calamus)

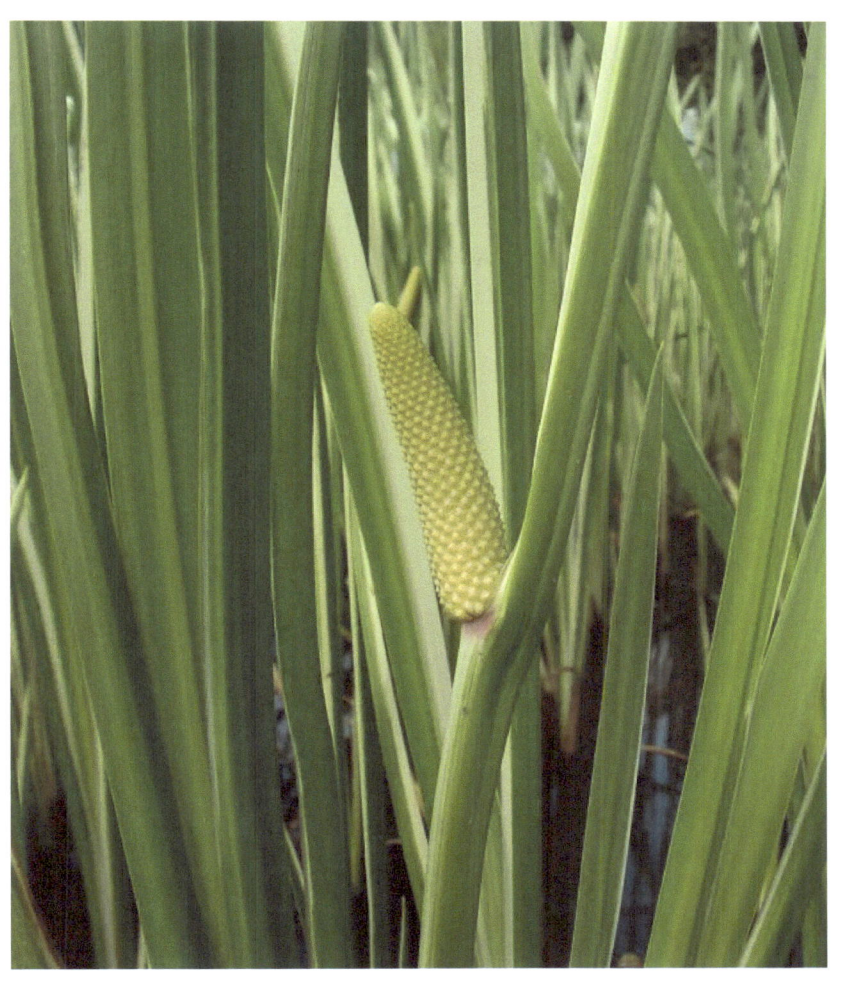

General

The scented leaves and more strongly scented rhizomes have traditionally been used medicinally and to make fragrances, and the dried and powdered rhizome has been used as a substitute for ginger, cinnamon and nutmeg. The dry rootstock yields a yellow coloured, aromatic, antiseptic volatile oil on steam-distillation.

Calamus oil is an acknowledged nerve-stimulant, helpful in mental concentration exercises. The oil is effective against a host of ailments such as gastritis and various skin diseases due to its antiseptic properties.

Profile

Botanical Name : Acorus calamus

Family : Araceae

Appearance : A marshy, fragrant herb. Leaves - simple, alternate, linear, glossy bright green. Flowers - fragrant, pale green on a stump. Fruit - a 3 celled fleshy capsule. Rootstock - pinkish brown, white and spongy inside.

Medicinal Parts : Rootstock (rhizome)

Distribution: Probably indigenous to India or Arabia, Acorus calamus is now found across Europe, southern Russia, northern Asia Minor, southern Siberia, China, Indonesia, Japan, Burma, Sri Lanka, Australia, as well as southern Canada and the northern United States.

Ailments and Cure

Colic, Flatulence - Burn a piece of the root till charred. Mix with a little castor (or coconut) oil and apply over lower abdomen.

Cough - Paint a smooth coat of castor oil over root-stock and then char it over a flame. Store the ash from charred root. Mix 2 pinches of this ash with an equal quantity of honey and administer in 3 doses a day.

5. <u>Castor</u>

(Ricinus communis)

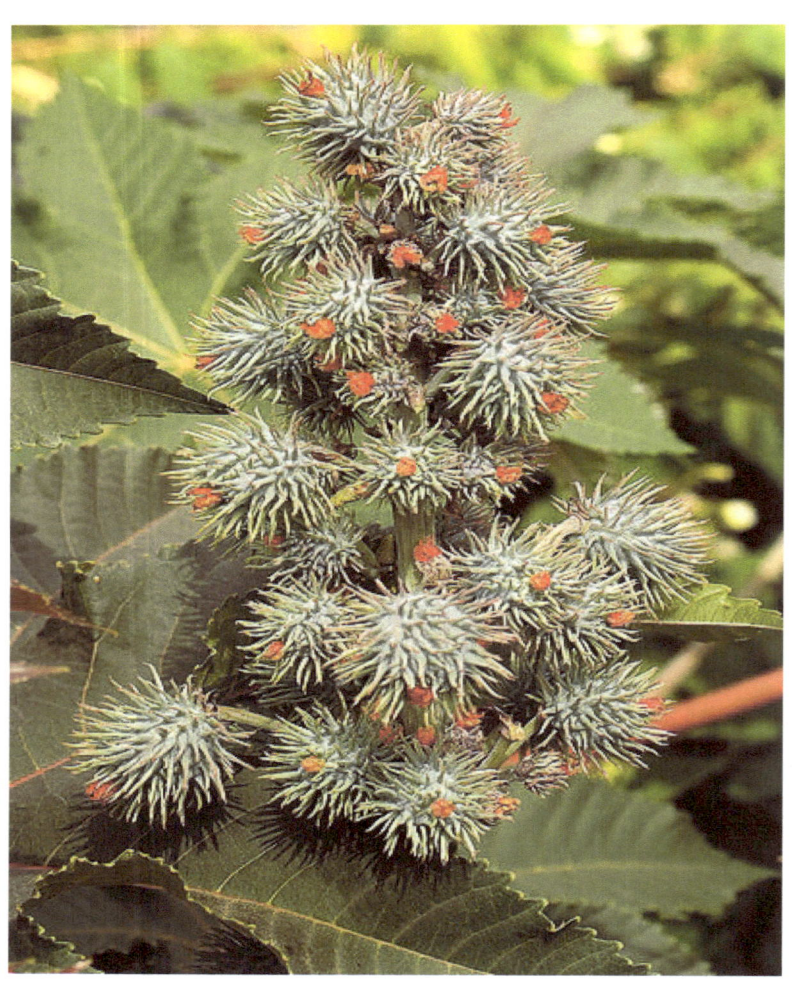

General

Castor seed is the source of castor oil, which has a wide variety of uses. The seeds contain between 40% and 60% oil that is rich in triglycerides, mainly ricinolein. The seed contains ricin, a toxin, which is also present in lower concentrations throughout the plant.

Medicinally, castor oil is a strong purgative.

Profile

Botanical Name : Ricinus communis

Other Species : white seeded castor, pale seeded castor

Family : Euphorbiaceae

Appearance : A tree like shrub, herbaceous, 3 to 10 feet tall. Leaves - palm like. Fruit - spiny capsule. Seeds - glossy.

Medicinal Parts : Leaves, seeds, roots, oil from seeds

Distribution: Castor is indigenous to the southeastern Mediterranean Basin, Eastern Africa, and India, but is widespread throughout tropical regions.

Ailments and Cure

Flatulence - Coat the leaves with castor oil and warm it over a flame. Apply these warm leaves over abdomen.

6. <u>Coriander</u>

(Coriandrum sativum)

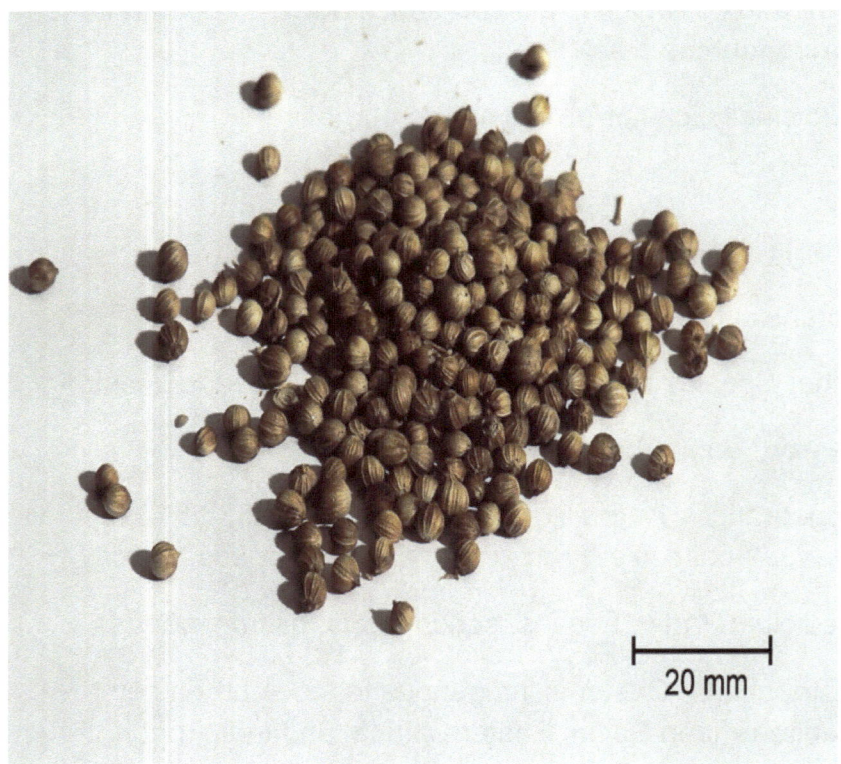

20 mm

General

Coriander (Coriandrum sativum), also known as cilantro,
Chinese parsley or dhania is an annual herb, well known for
its carminative and cooling properties.

Both leaves of coriander and its seeds are effective household remedy for many ailments.

Profile

Botanical Name : Coriandrum sativum

Family : Apiaceae

Appearance : Aromatic herb with dissected leaves.

Medicinal Parts : Leaves, seeds

Distribution : Coriander is native to regions spanning from southern Europe and North Africa to southwestern Asia.

Ailments and Cure

Bed-wetting – Fry 1 tsp crushed coriander seeds in a cast-iron skillet until they are lightly burnt. Mix in 1 tsp each pomegranate flowers, ground sesame seeds and gum acacia. Add brown sugar to equal the amount of powdered herbs. Take 1 tsp at bedtime.

7. <u>Garlic</u>

<u>*(Allium sativum)*</u>

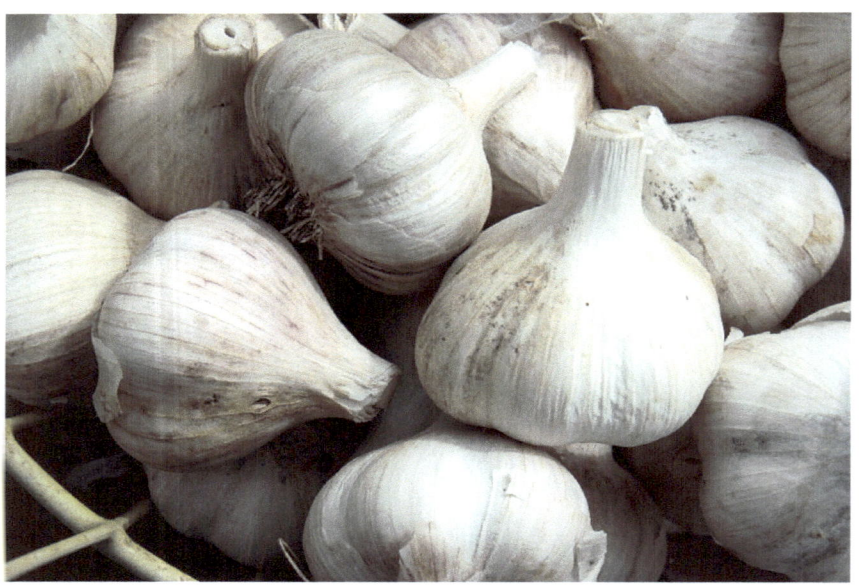

General

Garlic is held in high esteem for its medicinal use for over six thousand years. It is considered a powerful rejuvenating herb. It acts as a stimulant and anti-bacterial.

Garlic is widely used around the world for its pungent flavor as a seasoning or condiment.

Profile

Botanical Name : Allium sativum

Family : Liliaceae

Appearance : Herb of the onion family. The bulb consists of 6-35 bulblets called cloves enclosed in a white, glistening, transparent jacket.

Medicinal Parts : Bulb

Distribution : Garlic is native to central Asia. Now, it is grown globally - China, India, South Korea, Egypt, Russia, and the United States.

Ailments and Cure

Bronchitis in children – Mix 1 tsp juice of garlic and 3 tsp honey. Let the child eat a small amount three times a day.

Cold, phlegm – 2 garlic cloves crushed and boiled in a cup of water along with ½ tsp turmeric powder. Filter and rub the chest and throat with it.

8. <u>Haritaki</u>

(Terminalia chebula)

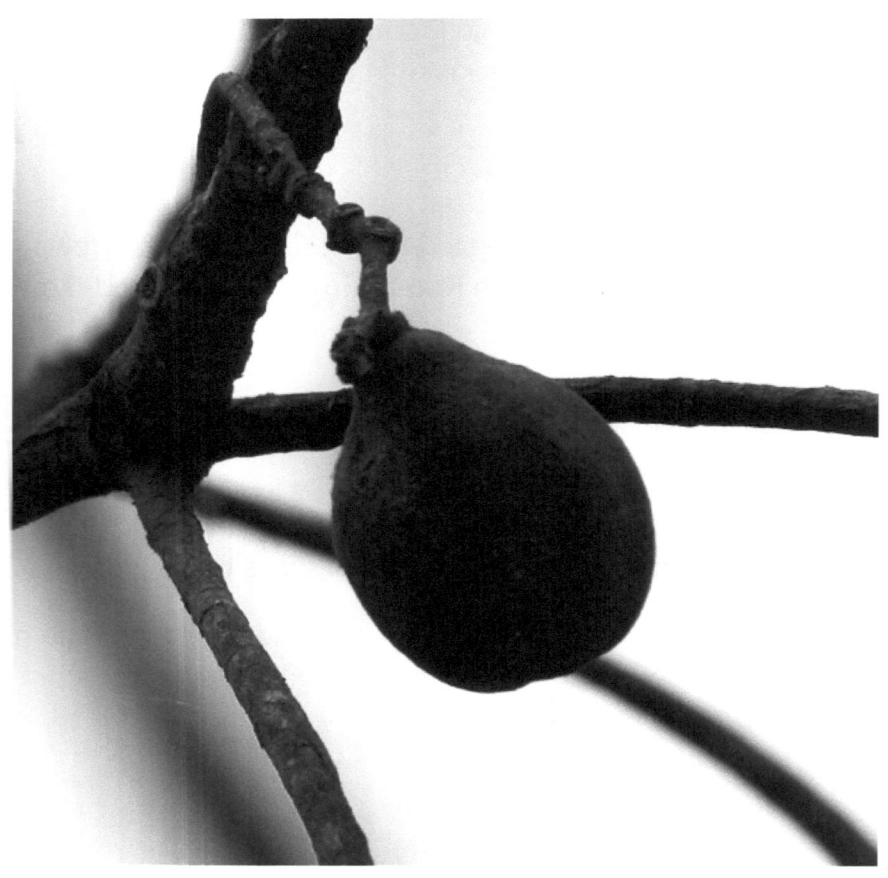

General

Haritaki, an indigenous tree of the Indian subcontinent has been in medicinal use for long. It is considered effective in many ailments. This tree yields smallish, ribbed and nut-like fruits which are picked when still green and then used for treatments.

The dry nut's peel is used to cure asthma. The bark/peel of the nut is placed in the cheek. Although the material does not dissolve, the resulting saliva, bitter in taste, is believed to have medicinal qualities to cure asthma.

Profile

Botanical Name : Terminalia chebula

Family : Combretaceae

Appearance : Tree with dark brown bark. Leaves - simple, opposite, shiny. Flowers - small cream coloured. Fruits - an ellipsoidal drupe, 5-angled, 4x2.5 cm.

Medicinal Parts : Rind of the fruit (raw or dried). Note - seeds should never be used.

Distribution: Native to southern Asia from India and Nepal east to southwestern China (Yunnan), and south to Sri Lanka, Malaysia and Vietnam. Found mainly in deciduous forests up to 1000m.

Ailments and Cure

Mumps - Grind the fruit with a little water into a thick, smooth paste and apply on the affected areas.

9. <u>Nutmeg</u>

(Myristica fragrans)

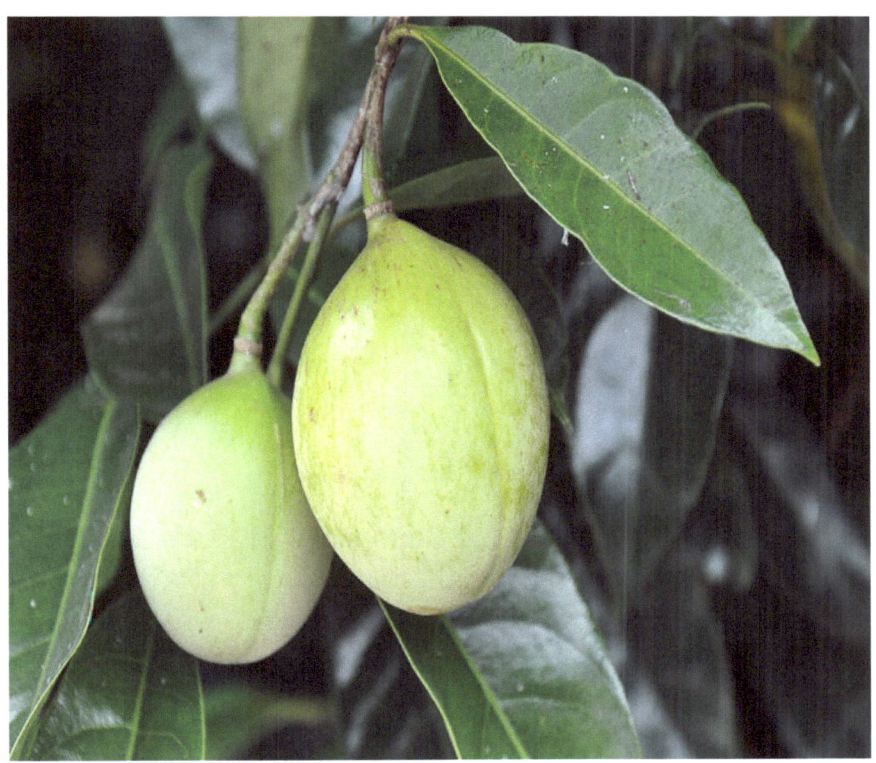

General

The nutmeg tree is important for two spices derived from the fruit: nutmeg and mace. Nutmeg is the seed of the tree while mace is the dried "lacy" reddish covering or aril of the seed.

Nutmeg is aromatic and bitter. It is considered a stimulant tonic. Its volatile constituents, particularly myristicin, is responsible for its pharmacological as well as toxic effects.

Profile

Botanical Name : Myristica fragrans

Family : Myristicaceae

Appearance : Small evergreen tree with smooth greyish-brown bark. Leaves alternate, smooth, dark green. Flowers small, creamy yellow, inconspicuous and uni-sexual. Fruit is peach like. Fruit cover is hard, encasing a soft brown seed smelling like varnish.

Medicinal Parts : Kernel, aril, oil.

Distribution: Indigenous to the Banda Islands in the Moluccas (or Spice Islands) of Indonesia, is also grown in Penang Island in Malaysia and the Caribbean, especially in Grenada. It also grows in Kerala, a state in southern India.

Ailments and Cure

Irritability in children – Rub a nutmeg lightly against a smooth grinding stone in milk and feed children who cry out at night without any apparent reasons. Dosage : 1 pinch. (Caution: Prolong use to be avoided as it may cause addiction.)

10. <u>Peepul</u>

(Ficus religiosa)

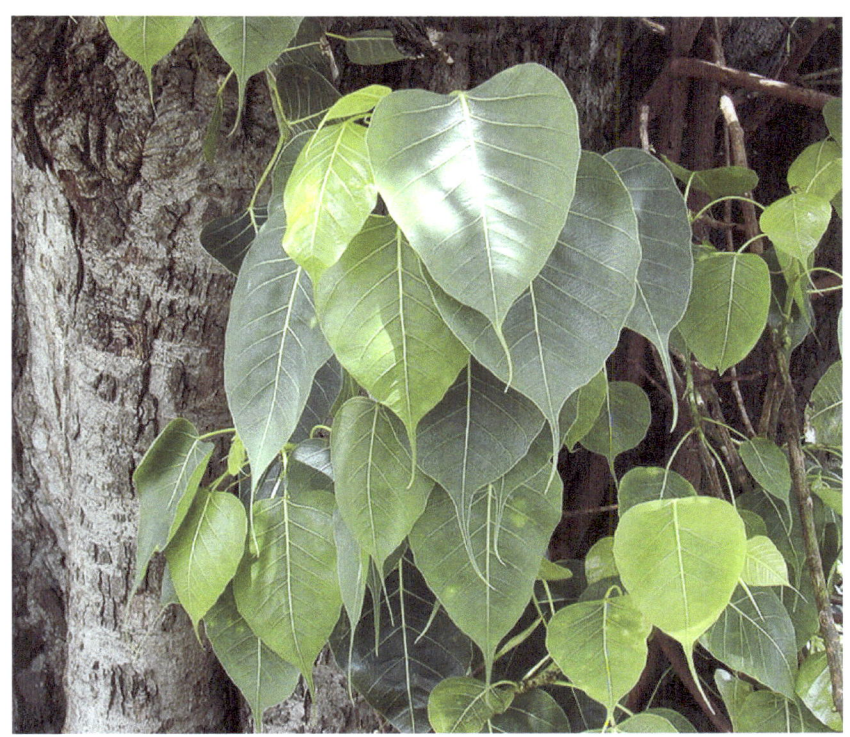

General

The peepul tree is considered sacred by the followers of Hinduism, Jainism and Buddhism.

The peepul is a large dry season-deciduous or semi-evergreen tree up to 30 meters tall and with a trunk diameter of up to 3 meters. The leaves are cordate in shape with a distinctive extended tip; they are 10–17 cm long and 8–12 cm broad, with a 6–10 cm petiole. The fruit is a small fig 1-1.5 cm diameter, green ripening to purple.

Profile

Botanical Name : Ficus religiosum, Urostigma religiosum

Family : Moraceae

Appearance : Large tree with characteristic milky exudate; deltoid peppery leaves with very long petioles which produce rustling music at the slightest puff of wind. Bark is smooth and light gray in colour, peeling off in bits and patches. Flowers - inconspicuous and colourless. Fruits - green and smooth when unripe, purple when ripe.

Medicinal Parts : Bark, leaf buds, fruits.

Distribution : Native to India, Bangladesh, Nepal, Pakistan, Sri Lanka, southwest China and Indochina.

Ailments and Cure

Mumps - Take a peepul leaf. Smear it with ghee and warm slightly over a naked flame. Use as bandage when lukewarm on the affected parts.

11. <u>Saffron</u>

(Crocus sativus)

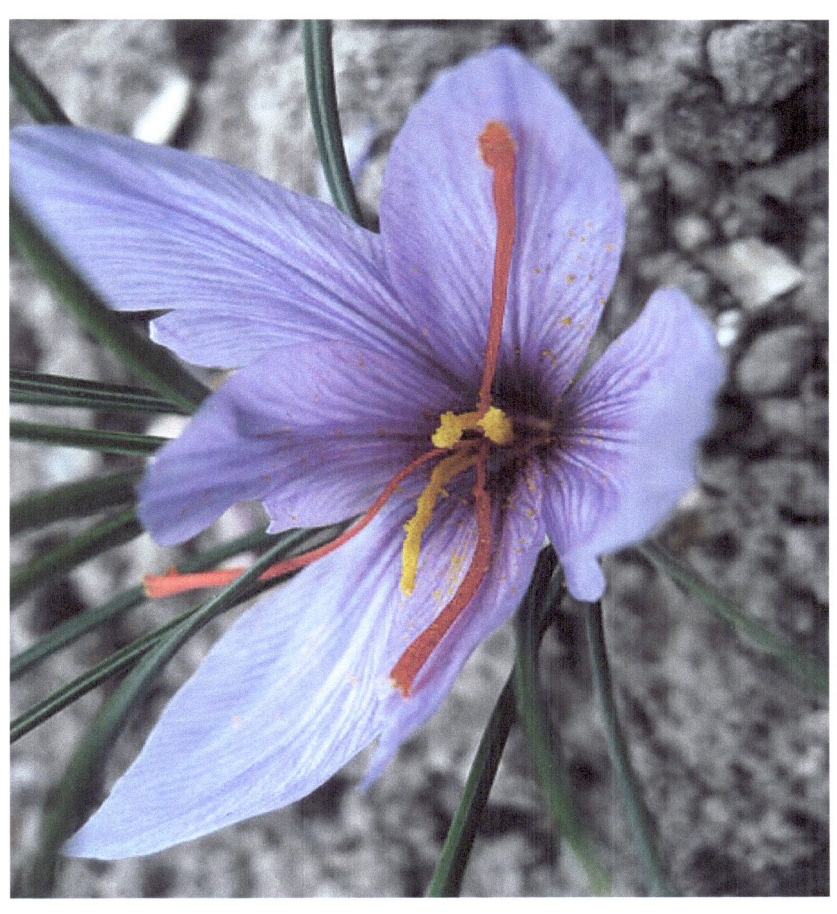

General

Saffron is a spice derived from the flower of Crocus sativus, commonly known as the saffron crocus. Commercial saffron consists of the tiny, dried stigmas and styles of flowers.

Profile

Botanical Name : Crocus sativus

Family : Iridaceae

Appearance : A bulbous perennial, saffron grows to 20–30 cm and bears up to four flowers, each with three vivid crimson stigmas, which are each the distal end of a carpel.

Medicinal Parts : The dried stigmas and tops of the styles.

Distribution : Saffron is native to Greece or Southwest Asia and was first cultivated in Greece. It slowly propagated throughout much of Eurasia and was later brought to parts of North Africa, North America, and Oceania.

Ailments and Cure

Cold and phlegm in children – Grind ½ tsp saffron in milk (preferably human milk) and apply on nose, head, cheeks etc.

12. <u>Sesame</u>

(Sesamum indicum)

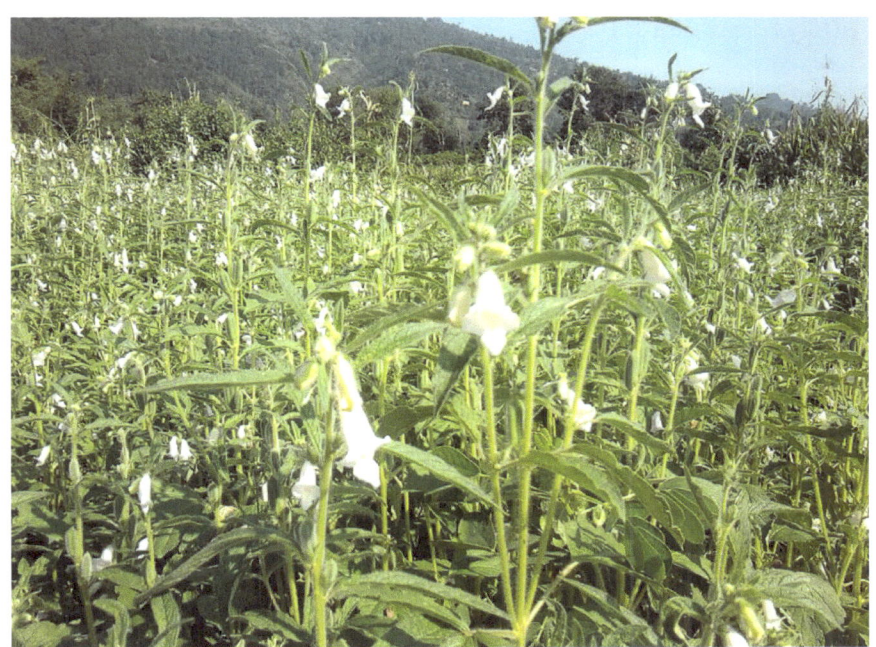

General

Sesame is a flowering plant and is cultivated for its edible seeds, which grow in pods.

Sesame seed is considered to be the oldest oilseed crop known, domesticated well over 5000 years ago. Sesame is very drought-tolerant. It has been called a survivor crop, with an ability to grow where most crops fail.

Profile

Botanical Name : Sesamum indicum

Family : Pedaliaceae

Appearance : Tall, erect, annual herb. Leaves ovate, grow alternately on the stem and are deeply veined. Flowers whitish yellow. Fruit is a two shelled pod which burst open when seeds are ripe. Seeds vary in color from yellowish white to black.

Medicinal Parts : Seeds, oil.

Distribution: It is widely naturalized in tropical regions around the world. Burma, India, and China account for 50 percent of global production.

Ailments and Cure

Bed-wetting – Fry 1 tsp crushed coriander seeds in a cast-iron skillet until they are lightly burnt. Mix in 1 tsp each pomegranate flowers, ground sesame seeds and gum acacia. Add brown sugar to equal the amount of powdered herbs. Take 1 tsp at bedtime.

Phlegm – Heat 1 tsp garlic in 3 tsp sesame oil. Rub this preparation on the chest and throat.

13. <u>Shatavari</u>

(Asparagus racemosus)

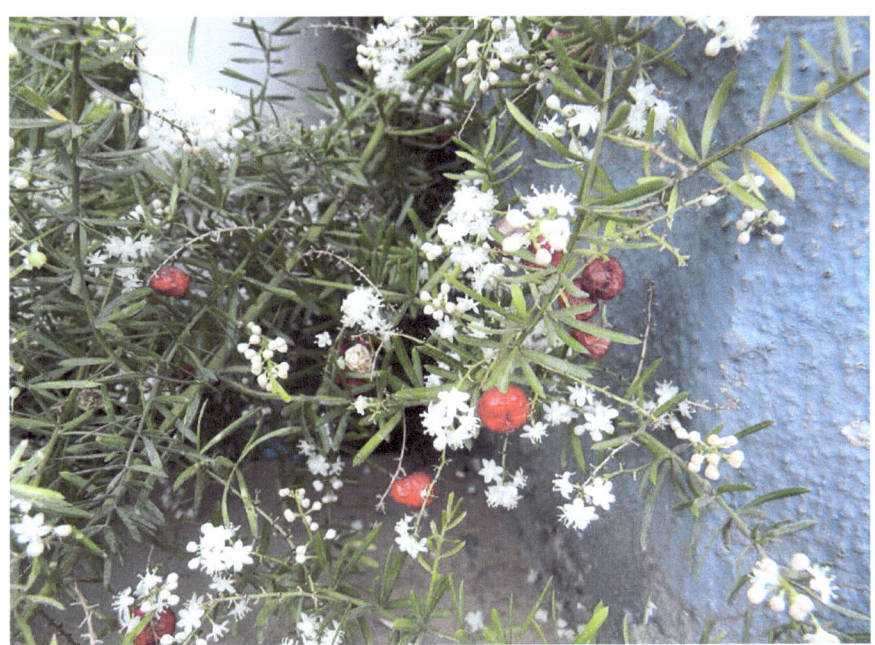

General

Shatavari is a perennial plant, generally cultivated for food; may be found wild around gardens and wastelands. It grows one to two meters tall and prefers to take root in gravelly, rocky soils high up in piedmont plains, at 1,300 - 1,400 meters elevation.

Shatavari is believed to improve physical as well as mental performance by slowing down the aging process. It is widely used in treatment of many ailments.

Profile

Botanical Name : Asparagus racemosus

Family : Liliaceae

Appearance : The short, horizontal rootstock has long, thick roots and sends up young shoots, used as a vegetable. What looks like leaves on the stem and branches are actually filiform branches which are clustered in the axis of the scaly inconspicuous leaves. Flowers - greenish white. Fruit - a red berry containing black seed.

Medicinal Parts : Root, young shoots, seeds.

Distribution: Found throughout Sri Lanka, India and the Himalayas.

Ailments and Cure

Mumps - Grind shatavari and fenugreek seeds together in equal quantities in sufficient water into a fine paste. Apply on the affected areas.

Some Important Guidelines

1. Preparation

When the herb is extremely bitter, sour, astringent or in powdered form, it can be mixed with honey, jaggery, sugar, candy etc.

2. Dosage

The quantity of dose can vary from one person to another based on individual age, physical build, and reaction of patient to a particular formulation.

The dosage prescribed in this book is meant for fully grown and mature patients. The dose should be increased/decreased for each patient keeping in mind individual patient's constitution.

3. Effectiveness

The contents of a herbal plant part varies widely due to factors such as climate, altitude, latitude, soil type, nutrition, temperature, relative humidity, time of plucking, packaging, storage etc. Hence the effectiveness of herb for treating an ailment may vary in different cases.

Patient needs to keep in mind this inherent weakness of herbal effectiveness, and be prepared to continue the treatment for a little longer time.

Other Books That May Interest You

Herbs That Cure:

Anaemia
Asthma
Bad Breath
Bronchitis
Constipation
Diabetes
Diarrhoea
ENT Problems
Fatigue
Flatulence
Genito-Urinal disorders
Haemorrhoids
Hair Loss
Heart Problems
Insomnia
Joints Pain
Leucoderma
Obesity
Pimples
Psoriasis
Rheumatism
Sexual Debility
Skin Diseases
Stomach Disorders
Toothache
Venereal Diseases
Wrinkles

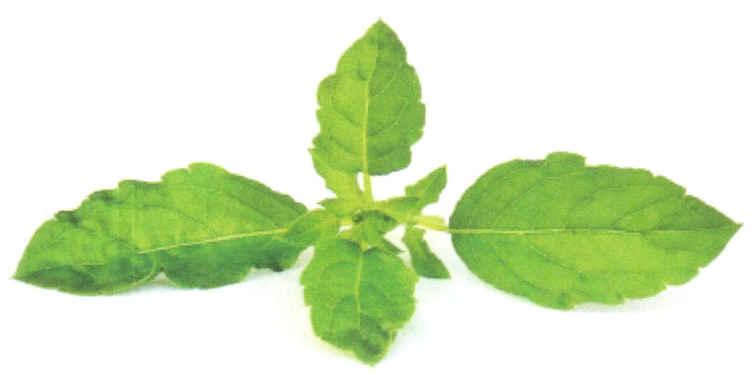